YOUR KNOWLEDGE HAS VALUE

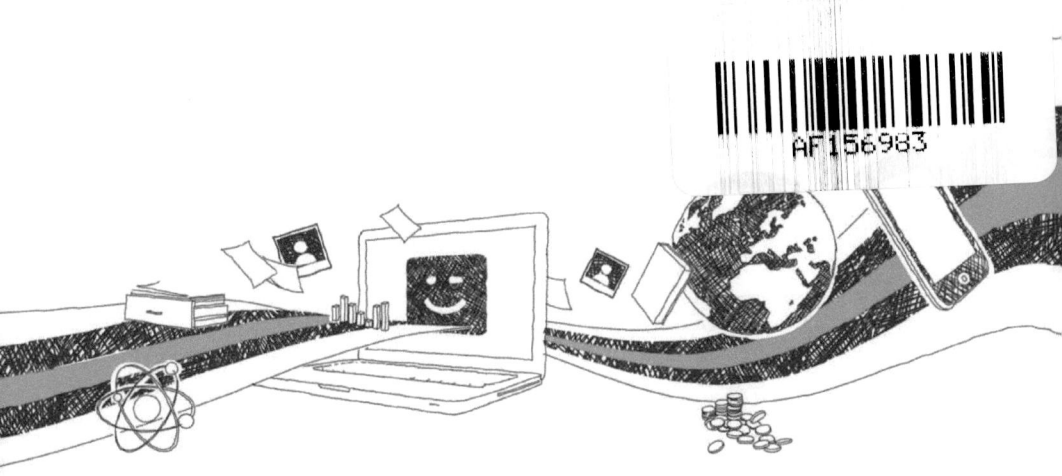
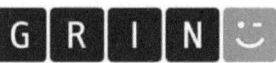

Bibliographic information published by the German National Library:

The German National Library lists this publication in the National Bibliography; detailed bibliographic data are available on the Internet at http://dnb.dnb.de .

Imprint:

Copyright © 2017 GRIN Verlag
Print and binding: Books on Demand GmbH, Norderstedt Germany
ISBN: 9783668660557

This book at GRIN:

https://www.grin.com/document/385881

Tamene Bayisa

Review on Effect of Feeding Dairy Cow with Protected Fat and Protein on milk Yield and its Composition

GRIN Verlag

GRIN - Your knowledge has value

Since its foundation in 1998, GRIN has specialized in publishing academic texts by students, college teachers and other academics as e-book and printed book. The website www.grin.com is an ideal platform for presenting term papers, final papers, scientific essays, dissertations and specialist books.

Visit us on the internet:

http://www.grin.com/

http://www.facebook.com/grincom

http://www.twitter.com/grin_com

JIMMA UNIVERSITY COLLEGE OF AGRICULTURE AND VETERINARY MEDICINE

Review on Effect of Feeding Dairy Cow with Protected Fat and
Protein on milk Yield and its Composition

Prepared by: Tamene Bayisa Daba

*Submitted to the Jimma University College of Agriculture and Veterinary Medicine Department
of Animal science, in fulfillment of the Requirements for the Course Current Topic in Animal
Production*

Jimma, Ethiopia
December, 2017

Acknowledgment

God, the Almighty, helped me to pass through tough times that cannot be forgotten in every corner of my life. Had it not been the will of God, nothing would have been possible. So, I would like to thanks GOD. I would like to extend my thanks to advisor Mohammed Aliyi (MSc) , whom I found to be helpful in guiding and commenting me by devoting his time to make me accomplish this paper.

Contents

List of table

List of Abrivation

AP-CLA,	Amide Protected Conjugeted Lenolic Acid
CLA	Conjugated Linoleic Acid
DM	Dry Mater
EE	Ether Extract (Fcm) Fat Correct Milk
DM I	Dry Mater Intake
FCMY	Fat Correct Milk Yield
IVDMD	*In Vitro* Dry Matter Digestible
LE-CLA,	Lipid-Encapsulated Conjugated Linoleic Acid
N E B	Negative Energy balance
NDF	Nutral detergent Fiber
OM	Organic Matter
TGP	Total Gas Production
RUP	Rumen Undegradable Protein

Abstract

Objective of this review is focus on effect of feeding protected fat and protected protein on milk yield and its composition and how these nutrients are protected . Many researchers in this review investigate that the responses are highly dependent on the type of fat and protein supplement and the stage of lactation. A higher milk response was observed with saturated than with unsaturated fat supplements . Diet with added fat increase milk production compared with a control diet without added fat in cows. Feeding of bypass fat resulted in significant increase in milk yield and Fat Corrected Milk yield particularly in early lactation . The source of Protected fat are (origin (animal, plant, processed or whole oilseeds, calcium salts) and Cereal Grains such as corn , wheat , Barly , oil seeds, sun flower, cotton seed, soybeans and canola) . The supplementation of protected protein in the diets of lactating animals increases the milk yield due to proportionate increase in the supply of amino acids to the host postruminally Milk yield in cows fed protected methionine for the whole experimental period was numerically higher than in cows of the other groups. However, the difference was not statistically significant .At the centeral high land of Ethiopia the Treatment of shredded wheat and barley straw with urea, molasses, salt and water prior to feeding is a technology that should be considered . Cows with excessive body tissue mobilisation at this stage may take up to 20 weeks to regain a positive energy balance status .

Key words milk yield ,composition ,protected fat , protien protected

1.Introduction

In tropical countries, the majority of livestock subsist on poor quality native grasses, crop residues and agro- industrial byproducts. Therefore, high yielding and genetically improved dairy animals has big challenge to provide the essential nutrients for meeting metabolic requirements and sustaining milk production . So many scholars and researchers reported that Traditionally ,cereal grains have been used to increase the energy density of diet in the ration of high producing dairy cattle which adversely affect the dry matter in take depresses fiber digestion and results in milk fat depression syndrome (Shelke et al.;2012). In designing protein and/or amino acid supplements for lactating cows in, it is essential to formulate supplements with an amino acid content that is complementary to microbial protein, which is considered to be the best available source of essential amino acids for milk synthesis (Gulati et, al., 2008). Similarly   in high producing dairy animals, specially during early lactation , the amount of energy and protein required for maintainance of body tissues and milk production often exceeds the amount of energy available   from diet which results negative energy balance (Taylor et al ,2003) . The research conducted by Strusińska ,et al., (2006) at University of Warmia and Mazuria, Olsztyn, Poland perform experiment on Holstein-Frisian cows during the first 120 days of lactation Megapro Plus supplementation of a diet with a reduced (to 3%) rapeseed meal content in concentrate (group 2) resulted increased unsaturation milk fat, and positive changes in the fatty acid composition, reflected by improved health properties of milk. According to Shelke et.al. ; (2012) high yield can achieved from the early lactating improved cows were fed according to the nutrient requirement with high energy diet. Fat supplementation affects milk fat percentage and composition in different ways. Fat feeding may have negative effects on rumen fiber digestion and decrease acetic and butyric acid (precursors of short- and medium-chain FA in milk) production, affecting de novo fat synthesis in mammary gland. According to Tekebe et al (2014) reported that Urea Molasses Multi-nutrient Blocks fulfill several demands and should therefore be considered in strategies which aim to improve the nutritional situation of dairy cows in several regions of Ethiopia . According to Hassen A et al , (2010) Supplemental feeds such as the by products of grain and oil seed mills are fed to livestock especially when there is shortage of feed. Farmers in high altitude zone, especially those around the peri-urban areas, utilize by-products of grain for lactating crossbred cows. By- products of oil seeds secured through purchase from the local market are mixed with straw and other local supplements such as the spent brewer's grains from the local manufacture of *"atela"* to feed livestock especially cross-bred dairy cows in Ethiopia.

Objective

To review effect of protected fat and protein on milk yield and milk composition And how to protect protein feed

2. Literature Review

2.1. Effect of feeding Dairy cows with protected fat on milk yield

Application of supplements of protected fats and polyenoic fatty acids of vegetable origin in a diet of different age and productive groups of cattle stimulates metabolism in the animals, increases their productivity and improves quality of milk (Pavkovych et al 2015) . Dietary fat, that resists biolysis and biohydrogenation in rumen by rumen microorganisms, but gets digested in lower digestive tract, is known as bypass fat or rumen protected fat (inert fat) (Naik,*2011)*. Supplementation of fat to pasture based system appears to increase milk production by dairy cows grazing high-quality pastures such as (Perennial rye grass, Red clover, White clover, Alfalfa,in cool season) and Cereal Grains such as corn , wheat , Barly , oil seeds, sun flower, cotton seed, soybeans and canola) (Muller, 2003) and by products of cereal grains and oilseed during feed shortage for lactating cows in Ethiopia (Hassen A et al 2010). The responses are highly dependent on the type of fat supplement and the stage of lactation. The percentage of fat in , Cotton seed 20%, Soy bean 18.8%, sun flower 44.4% , canola 40.2%, saturated fatty acids (SFA) cotton seed 26%, soybean 15%, sunflower 12%, palm oil 51% ,canola 06% and unsaturated fatty acids (USFA) cottonseed 74%,Soybean 85%,Sunflower 88%and palm 49% of different oil seeds in ration of Dairy cows are reviewed by (Naik ,2013). A higher milk response was observed with saturated than with unsaturated fat supplements . The effect of supplementation of dietary fat on milk and FCM production was related to the degree of saturation of the fat supplement and to the stage of lactation. Supplementation with unsaturated Fatty Acid sources did not significantly increase milk or FCM production where as both parameters were increased by saturated FA supplements.

Mid-lactation cows had higher milk yield response to fat supplementation but a lower production of FCM than early-lactation cows. Maximum milk production response to fat supplementation may not be achieved until cows are in a positive energy balance (Muller, 2003). The influence of varying levels of bypass fat on the milk yield and its composition of lactating crossbred cows is examined lactating cows The dry matter intake was not affected by feeding different levels of fat in contrastan addition of dietary fat, which increases the energy density of the cows' diet, may limit and/or shorten Negative Energy Balance (NEB) in early lactated dairy cows. because the impact of dietary fat is influenced by the sourceof fat, method of processing, amount of fat included in the diet, and stage of lactation (Kirovski et al, 2015) . this shows that at day 86 of lactation, 5.46 ± 0.32 urea and 3.26 ± 0.09 glucose concentrations were significantly lower in the palm oil-supplemented compared to the control Urea 6.58 ± 0.38 and Glucose 3.76 ± 0.06 respectively ; at day 58, 3.25 ± 0.04 Ca concentration was significantly higher in the palm oil-supplemented compared to the control group 3.07 ± 0.06 and at day 86, cholesterol concentration was significantly higher in the experimental 5.93 ± 0.39 compared to 4.45 ± 0.31thecontrol group . This is Similar to the result presented by (Sirohi et al.,2010)Feeding of bypass fat resulted in significant increase in milk yield and FCM yield particularly in early lactation. Milk yield and FCM yield was increased by 15.61% and 24.01% in bypass fat fed group over the control group.

Effects of dietary lipids on milk production:- most researchers indicate that addition of dietary fat had a positive effect on energy metabolism by decreasing hepatic lipid and increasing liver glycogen content in transition dairy cows (Patton et al.,2004) . Simalrly Feeding bypass fat at the rate of 100-150 g day-1 to high yields during the transition period (10 days before and 90 days after calving) could help improving their milk production and reproduction efficiency (Garg et al., 2008) . Diets with added fat generally increase milk production compared with a control diet without added fat in cows. In cows, the increase is greater when given encapsulated animal fats or calcium salts of palm oil FA and when the saturation degree is higher (Martínez et al.,2013) . similarly study reported that the development of process of encapsulation of lipids in formaldhyde treated protein allows the feeding of large ruminant without adversely affecting rumen fermentation. Through the supplementation of by pass fat not only energy intake but also possible to increase unsaturated fatty acid in the milk (Garg et al ,2009) so during lactation stage, dairy cows require a lot of energy to produce milk. Energy can be increased either by higher dry matter intake (DMI), greater energy density in the diet or both. However, there is a limit to DMI. Once the limit is reached, what is needed is to raise the energy density of the dairy cow's diet. Therefore, the goal is to increase the energy intake without consuming more feed volume(InfluxLipds ,2017).

Table 1 effect of feeding Dairy cow with protected fat on milk yield

Item	Group 1	Group 2	Group 3	Types of supplement feed	Authors
	Mean $\pm$SD	Mean $\pm$SD	Mean $\pm$SD		
Milk yield(kg/Day)	29.56$\pm$2.78	32.59$\pm$2.95	32.61$\pm$3.94	Haylage,Silag concentratedf at & protein,	Strunka et al ,2006
	12.38$\pm$0.34	13.20$\pm$0.41	13.20$\pm$0.31	Geen maize ,fodder and straw	Garg et al.;2009
	14.52$\pm$ 0.18	16.01$\pm$ 0.24	16.00$\pm$0.24	Wheatstraw,Concentrate mixiture and green Maize fodder and By pass totreatment	Kirovski et al (2015)
Milkyield(kg /Day	11.40$\pm$0.38	13.18$\pm$0.16	-	Corn silage-based diet, without palmoil for group 1 and with 300 g palm oil (Palm Fat) after parturition.	Sirohi,et al.;*2010*
(Day 30)	22.90 $\pm$ 0.90	21.88 $\pm$ 0.91	-		
(Day 58)	21.91 $\pm$ 0.97	23.33 $\pm$ 1.10	-		
(Day86)	20.96 $\pm$ 1.55	21.72 $\pm$ 1.49	-		

2.2. Effect of protectedfat on milk composition

According to *Martínez al et.,(2013)* Fat supplementation affects milk fat percentage and composition in different ways. the effect of milk composition fat supplementation on milk fat percentage was not different from zero. However, when the effects were separated by type of fat supplement, saturated FA sources increased milk fat percentage by 5.1% (3.50 to 3.68%), and unsaturated FA sources reduced milk fat percentage 8.0% (3.5 to 3.22%). Fat feeding may have negative effects on rumen fiber digestion and decrease acetic and butyric acid (precursors of short- and medium-chain FA in milk) production, affecting de novo fat synthesis in mammary gland. When fat is included in the ration, the uptake and direct incorporation of long-chain FA into Total Growth by the mammary gland are increased.

In addition   36% of the 25 comparisons, a significant increase in milk fat production was observed. Similar to the results found for milk fat percentage, milk fat yield was increased more by saturated fat supplements [+75.5 g/d (+9.3%)] than by unsaturated fat supplements . The overall effect of unsaturated fats on milk fat yield in grazing conditions was not different from zero and can be explained by the combination of a decrease in the milk fat concentration and an increase in milk production (Muller,2003).

Feeding fat for a longer period increased DMI, as did greater differences in the amount of soluble protein percentage of the diet between control and treatment diets (**Rabiee,et al,2012).**

According to **Lock et al , (2013)** Addition of fat to the diet can increase the concentration and yield of milk fat. This response however, is inconsistent and often related to the amount and type of fat being fed. Unsaturated fatty acids have the potential to affect the growth of some groups of rumen bacteria and inhibit fat synthesis in the mammary gland. On the other hand, saturated fatty acids (e.g. palmitic [C16:0] and stearic [C18:0] acids) are considered to be inert in the rumen and have not been implicated in milk fat depression (MFD).

Limitations of feeding fats to early lactation cows As a general rule of thumb, unsaturated fatty acids such as those found in canola oil are relatively toxic to the rumen microbes. This is especially true for forage-fibre digesting species. With that being said, this doesn't mean that canola oil or other types of unsaturated fatty acids should not be fed to dairy cows. Most rumen microbes have the ability to detoxify and reduce the toxic effect of unsaturated fats through a process called "bio-hydrogenation". However, large amount of unsaturated fatty acids (approximately 450g/head/d) can overwhelm this process,causing negative effects on the rumen microbial population. (*http://www2.luresext.edu/international/NutrConstraints.htm.*) According to Pavkovych et al (2015) proved that increasing the level of fats and fatty acids in the diets of cattle inhibits process of fiber digestion in the rumen , decrease digestion of organic matter in the fore stomach.

2.3. Sources of protected fat (By pass fat)

Corn oil for fatty acids derived from beef tallow and olive oil. However, it is unlikely that the protection afforded by these dietary fats is effectively with PUFA for esterification into phospholipids. No change occurred in composition of SFA . Instead, a major shift between linoleic acid and oleic acid occurred. data suggest that diets with high MUFA protect against the hepatotoxicity of acetaminophen by affecting the fatty acid composition of membrane phospholipids, thereby reducing susceptibility to free radical damage(Hwang et al.2011) . The addition of fat sources of different type and origin (animal, plant, processed or whole oilseeds, calcium salts) to the diet of ewes and goats generally increases milk fat content as opposed to dairy cows (*Martínez AL et al.2012*).Oilseeds contain polyunsaturated fatty acids, but they are slowly digested and the oil is gradually released into the rumen, thus allowing for saturation of the fatty acids and less chance of reduced fiber digestibility or milk fat depression (Chiba, 2014) . Plant oil supplements provide a dietary source of unsaturated fatty acids, but if changes in the ruminal VFA pattern and the reduce roughage intake is high then rumen microbial protien in milk fat yield (Bauman and Griinari ,2001) . The source of Oil seeds Cotton ,Soybean, Sunflowe ,Palm,Canola (Naik ,2013). The economic value of the energy from fat will be affected by market costs of other energy sources such as cereal grains and alternative uses of fats. Fat must be fed *in moderation* to dairy cattle. About 2% to 3% fat will be present from typical dietary ingredients, and initial levels of supplemental fat generally will be 1% to 3% of dietary DM for increasing energy concentration of diets or delivery of some specific FA another source of by pass fat (Pavkovych et al.; 2015)Supplements of calcium salts of fatty acids, made of sunflower, soybean, rape, flax and palm oils are the most effective in a diet of young animals and cattle.

According to Lock et al., (2013) Performance of lactating cows receiving rumen-protected supplements of AP-CLA, Amide Protected CLA supplement; CLA, conjugated linoleic acid; LE-CLA, lipid-encapsulated CLA supplement in milk yield and composition . similarly (Stephen and Emanuele ,2006) reviewed that Feeding CLA through the first 20 weeks of lactation reduced milk fat percentage by 12.5%. During this period, cows receiving CLA tended to produce almost 3 kg/d more milk . The resulting increase in milk yield offset the reductions in milk fat percentage and resulted in only a 7.5% reduction in milk fat yield

Table 2. The effect of protected fat in milk yield and its composition of cow

Supplementation	Effects on Milk Yield	Effects on Milk Components	Authors
dietary fat	At Mid-lactation cows had higher milk yield	Lower At Mid-lactation	Muller, 2003.
bypass fat	bypass fat increase in milk yield,early lactation	Increase FCM yield early lactation	Sirohi et al., 2010
Palmoil	higher milk yield in the experimental compared to the control	at day 86 of lactation, urea and glucose concentrations were significantly lower compared to the control group. cholesterol concentration was significantly higher in the experimental compared to the control (+Ve rumen characterics)	Kirovski et al., 2015
Bergafat Poweder from palmoil	Milk yield remained unaltered across all the treatments	percent milk fat increased The reason for lack of response in milk yield may be that our diets have not supplied an ample amount of bypass protein or the animals had already reached their maximum potential of production	Sarwa et al ,2003
Lipids,SFA	help improving their milk production and reproductionefficiency	Increase milk fat by supplementation of ruminally protected lipids	Garg et al., 2008
Diets with added fat	Increase milk production compared with	at supplementation on milk fat percentage was not different from zero.	Martínez al et.,2013
Protected fat	Improve Milk yield (Highyieldingcows early lact)	reproductive efficiency and this strategic approach is economical for milk production at field condition	Gowda et al ,2012

supplement by Haylage , Silag concentrated fat & protein, Kirovski1,et al (2015) supplement by corn silage-based diet, without palm oil supplementation

Table 3 Performance of lactating cows receiving rumen-protected supplements of AP-CLA, CLA ; CLA,; LE-CLA, CLA supplement in milk yield and composition

Variable	Control	AP-CLA	LE-CLA	SEM	Probability	Authors
DMI, kg/d	30.6	31.6	30.4	0.9	0.50	Perfield *et al.*, 2004
DMI, kg/d	23.8	23.1	22.1	22.0	0.12	(Lock et al , 2013)
	40.5	42.6	42.7	3.5	0.32	Perfield *et al.*, 2004
	36.9	37.3	35.8	34.8	0.44	(Lock et al , 2013)
Milk fat, %	3.23[a]	2.37[b]	2.34[b]	0.15	<0.001	Perfield *et al.*, 2004
	3.37	3.86	3.32	2.61	0.03	(Lock et al , 2013)
Milk fat yield, kg/d	1.27[a]	1.00[b]	0.99[b]	0.08	<0.001	Perfield *et al.*, 2004
	1,249	1,436	1,184	911	0.02	(Lock et al , 2013)
Milk protein yield, kg/d	1.00[b]	1.06[a]	1.09[a]	0.02	<0.02	Perfield *et al.*, 2004
10,12 CLA in milk fat, %	<0.01[b]	0.08[a]	0.09[a]	0.01	<0.001	Perfield *et al.*, 2004)
9,11 CLA in milk fat, %	0.57[b]	0.83[a]	0.80[a]	0.05	<0.001	Perfield *et al.*, 2004

2.4. Effect of feeding Dairy cows with protected protein on milk yield

The increase in milk yield in lactating dairy with increasing the dietary level of Rumen Undegradable Proten (RUP) is due to an increase in DM I as well as the increased supply of metabolizable protein and amino acids (Gulati *et at., 2005*). The slight decrease in the protein content of milk from cows fed a diet supplemented with nitrogen fraction of true protein and whey protein observed by (Strusińska, 2006) . Similarly Suresh et al.,(2011) it was observed that the response of milk production increases up to 501-600g Undegradableprotien (UDP) intake and there after, the milk production stabilizes with the increasing UDP levels. It was established that UDP intake of 571 g/h/day is required to produce an average of 10 kg 4% FCM (84.2% of accuracy). Milk yield and FCM yield is increased with increasing the dietary level of RDP while keeping the RUP proportion constant in **cows (Kalscheur *et at.,* 2006).** Increased milk production in response to increasing the dietary RDP is the result of providing additional Nitrogen for ruminal microbial protein synthesis and greater microbial protein synthesis supports greater milk production. However, milk yield and FCM remained unaltered in cows fed increasing level of Rumen Degradable Protien as reported by (Reynal and Broderick, 2005). There was no significant effect of treatments on nutrient(methonin) intake. Milk yield in cows fed protected methionine for the whole experimental period (subgroup MM) was numerically higher than in cows of the other groups. However, the difference was not statistically significant (Kudrna,2009). Milk contains approximately 3.2 – 3.5% protein. thus a cow producing 25 kg milk per day secretes 800–900 g protein daily. cows have little ability to store protein in the body and so it must be supplied in the diet daily to maintain the milk yield. protein should be 15–18% of the total ration of a dairy cow depending on milk yield (Lusweti and Mwendia ,2012) .

2.5. Effect of feeding Dairy cow with protected protien on milk composition

milk contains approximately 3.2–3.5% protein. thus a cow producing 25 kg milk per day secretes 800–900 g protein daily. cows have little ability to store protein in the body 8 and so it must be supplied in the diet daily to maintain the milk yield. protein should be 15–18% of the total ration of a dairy cow depending on milk yield(Lukuyu,et al ,2012). High-producing cows (> 5 kg milk/100 kg BW) will likely to benefit form more bypass protein.

The lowest milk protein concentrations were observed in cows that did not receive any ruminally protected methionine at all (subgroup OO). The methionine supplementation marginally increased methionine concentration in milk Concentrations of 7 out of 11 amino acids were significantly higher in milk of cows fed protected methionine for the whole experiment than in cows fed the unsupplemented diet (subgroups MM and OO, respectively). Five of these amino acids (threonine, valine, leucine, isoleucine, and lysine) are generally regarded as essential for humans. Milk fat of cows fed the diet protien of group OO contained significantly less lauric acid than milk fat of other cows .No other significant changes in the fatty acid profile of milk fat were During the first 120 days of lactation, the mean daily milk yield recorded in cows fed a diet supplemented with Megapro was by 3.03 kg (group 2) and 3.05 kg (group 3) higher than in the control group (increase by 10.3%). FCM yield increased by 15.5% and 12.1%,respectively, in comparison with group1. A higher dry matter energy concentration in the diet for group 2 allowed to increase milk fat content by 7.8% (4.23 vs. 4.56%), but it was accompanied by a slight decrease in the levels of milk protein (3.07 vs. 3.01%) and solids- non-fat , as compared with group 1 (control). The feeding of high levels of supplemental energy and protein in dairy cow diet (group 3) was characterized by slightly higher concentrations of fat (by 2.6%) and dry matter, and a lower protein level (by approx. 2%), in comparison with group 1 (statistically non-significant differences). Due to higher milk production in group 1 and 2, mean daily yields of major milk components were highly significantly or significantly higher than their yields recorded in the control group was observed (Strusińska, 2006) .

Dairy cow treated under experimental group fed with protected protein supplement at one month from stage of lactation significantly increase average daily milk yield and control groups are the same stage with the experimental group. However, the milk yield was apparently more after one month of lactation in all the treatment groups compared to control group (Shankare,et al., 2013) . similar to this According to Garg el al., (2005) feeding formaldehyde treated rapeseed meal increase not only milk yield but also increase fat percent in treatment group.According toMin et al., (2003) Moderate concentrations of condensed tannin (CT) can be used to increase the efficiency of protein digestion; however the effects are not the same for all Condensed tannin, but rather depend upon the concentration and structure of the CT. According to Kudrnaet al.,(2009) Milk yield in cows fed protected methionine for the whole experiment duration cows was higher and feed intake was lower than in cows of the other groups. The effect of protected methionine on milk yield was not, however, statistically significant. Effects of protected methionine on milk fat and protein were small and inconsistent.

Supplemental methionine significantly increased the methionine concentration in serum . while the methionine concentration in milk was not increased quite significantly . According to Mesfin et al., (2009) Treatment of crop residues with ammonia using fertilizer grade urea has received much attention, especially in Asia . Urea-ammonia treatment of straw is a technically effective and feasible on-farm technology to improve the nutritive value of fibrous crop residues. Feeding urea treated teff straw with bypass protein source was found to be an effective approach to maximize the utilization of locally available feed resources for better animal productivity during the dry season in mixed farming system of Ethiopia.

Table 4 Supplementation of dry season diets with UMMB

Traits	FogeraNonsupplemented	Fogerasupplemented	CN	CS	S_e
Milk offtake (l/day)	1.90[a]	2.35[b]	3.69[c]	4.95[d]	0.641
ECM offtake (l/day)	2.12[a]	2.78[b]	3.90[c]	5.42[d]	0.690
Milk fat (g/l of milk)	42.4[b]	47.5[c]	39.4[a]	42.1[b]	1.98
Milk protein (g/l of milk)	33.0[b]	33.2[b]	30.7[a]	30.8[a]	0.97
Milk total solids (g/l of milk)	133.4[b]	137.6[c]	123.4[a]	125.8[a]	3.62
Milk fat yield (g/day)	81[a]	112[b]	145[c]	209[d]	30.0
Milk protein yield (g/day)	63[a]	78[b]	113[c]	153[d]	19.2

Source :- Tekeba et al., 2013

Table 9 Ruminant diet containing rumen by pass proteins

Types of by pass proteins	Species	Response	Advantage	Ingridients
Form aldehydetreated soyabeansmeal	Lactating cow	Milk	Farther use of For aldehydeis not recomended	Not specified
Form aldehydetreated soyabeansmeal	Lactating cow	Milk	Increase production and milk protein	Diet were 60%concentrate, 22% corn silage 14% Alfaalfahay,4% beet palp(DM),
Heated soyabeanmeal	Lactating cow	Milk	Increase production	30% corn Silage,15% AlfaAlfa Hay,55% concentrate mix DM
Calcium salt treated soyabean meals	Dair cow	Milk	Increase production and milk fat	No information
Condense tannin in farage	Lactating Cows	In situ	Reduce protein digestion	Alfa Alfa and Bird foot trefoil,Rice bran, Casava wast, weat polard
Lignosulfonate SBM	In vitro	Rumen character stics	Reduce crude protein digestibility(15%),increase VFAconcentration(7%) , increase production	Diet contains (32%) corn silage , (19.8% Alfa Alfa grass hay)
Chemically treated SBM	Lactating Cows	Milk	Increased production	15%Vs CP Diet , 48.2 concentrate DMbasis

Source review of (Haryanto ,2014)

2.6. Economic aspect of feeding protected protein to Dairy cow

According to Garg et al .(2003) Economics of milk production on feeding protected Rapeseed meal was calculated and 1.0 kg protected Rapeseed meal as compared to unprotected resulted in increase average daily net income according to the data presented by (Tekebe ete al ,2014) concluded that supplementing dairy cows with UMMB during the dry season is basically a helpful measure to maintain a satisfactory level of production and to improve important economic traits of milk production in Ethiopia. Depending on the availability of UMMB, priority in supplementation should however be given to cows with a high genetic potential for milk production

3. Methods of protein protection

3.1.   Formaldehyde treatment

 It can be deduced that 1.5% formaldehyde treatment to mustard oil cake will be beneficial in increasing digestible undegradable protein in wheat straw containing diet without affecting the digestibility, but more studies are needed to validate the results under *in vivo* conditions. The result of this study might have implication in all other developing countries where the diet is based on straw and mustard cake, which is highly degradable in the rumen. Thus, protection of mustard cake by formaldehyde treatment may help in improving the protein supplementation of ruminants (Mahima et al,2015) . This is cormfirmed the reviewed of Haryanto, (2014) Protection of protein from microbial enzyme degradation can be carried out by linking the protein molecule to several chemicals such as formaldehyde . similar to this Shelke,et .al.,(2012**) revised that** treatments have also been used for the protection of proteins and for this formaldehyde treatment has been the most effective and feasible technology for manufacture of bypass protein. According to Khandaker et al.,(2012) supplementation of RDP from MOC enhances the intake, digestibility and microbial protein synthesis which ultimately increases utilization of low-quality feed resources that can be used for developing cost-effective feeding systems on a straw-based diet in tropical regions.

According to Haryanto, (2014) Manipulating dietary protein characteristics from readily degradable in the rumen to undegradable or partially degradable has the potency to improve the ruminant productivity; therefore further efforts to produce rumen bypass protein feedstuffs will open the possibility to increase farmers' economic benefit

3.2.   Heat treatment

Among the several methods which allow the escape of dietary protein from ruminal degradation, much of the work was carried out on heat treatment of highly degradable cakes. The problem with 'heat treatment' is that it may not be cost effective and moreover, it can also over-protect the protein (Shelke,et .al;.2012). Heat-treated soybeans may have greater protein bypass properties than unheated soybeans. (LeeI.Chiba, 2014)

3.3.   Using lateral flow device dipsticks

The method developed is based on a bone sedimentation procedure coupled with an Ethylediamine tetra acetic Acid (EDTA) digestion step in order to liberate the protected proteins which are covalently bound to mineral structures within the bone mineral cage. All the results using this method showed that the feed contaminated with ruminant material is detected at 0.1 to 0.2% levels (KaranamM,2011). The results confirmed the study of Protection of Animal Protein and Meat and Bone Meal in feeds produced in Poland between 2012 and 2013 (Weiner et al.,2015) that using microscopy technique enables detection of feed of animal origin constituents. Such as feathers, bones, fish bones, and scales were detected most frequently. The use of chemical reagents, especially cystinere agent and paraffin oil (embeding agent) improved the visualisation and identification of the constituents of animal origin in the samples examined.

4.Conclusion

Dietary fat that resists biolysis and biohydrogenation in rumen by rumen microorganisms, but gets digested in lower digestive tract, is known as bypass fat or rumen protected fat or inert fat . From available literature, it can be concluded that supplementation of bypass fat in the diet of dairy animals is very important to alleviate problems of negative energy balance without adversely affecting the dry matter intake and rumen fermentation. Supplementation of bypass fat gives additional benefit due to increase in milk yield and Fat Corrected Milk yield, efficiency of nutrient utilization, post partum recovery of reproductive performance of the dairy animals. However, long term trial in different seasons and at various locations to confirm this claim. Fat feeding may have negative effects on rumen fiber digestion and decrease acetic and butyric acid (precursors of short- and medium-chain FA in milk) production, affecting fat synthesis in mammary glan. The increase in milk yield and fat correct milk (FCM) in lactating ruminants with increasing the dietary level of RUP is due to an increase in DM I as well as the increased supply of metabolizable protein and amino acids.

It can be deduced that 1.5% formaldehyde treatment to mustard oil cake will be beneficial in increasing digestible undegradable protein in wheat straw containing diet without affecting the digestibility, but more studies are needed to validate the results under *in vivo* conditions. Supplementation of dairy cows with Formaldehydetreated soyabeansmeal , Heated soyabeanmeal, Calcium salt treated soyabean meals, Condense tannin in farage, Lignosulfonate SBM and Chemically treated SBM are protected protein that affect milk yield and its composition. Feeding of urea treated teff straw supplemented with a concentrate mixture containing linseed cake as a bypass protein source (slowly degradable N source) was found to be an economically viable and practical approach to maximize the utilization of locally available feed resources for better animal productivity during the dry season in mixed farming system in of Ethiopia.

5. Recommendation

- In Ethiopian country government must take in to consideration that training should be given for extension workers and experts about knowledge of protected fat and protein feeding to lactating cows .

- It is important train the farmers to ensure that the diet is still well balanced with carbohydrates, protein, water and mineral to support the health and normal activities of the resident microbes in the rumen.

- In Ethiopian Country there is no adequate conducted research regarding this review , so Further research is necessary to be find out the supplemental effect of the bypass fat on dairy animals feed various types of basal rations at different productive levels and stages of lactation

References

Kudrna, J V. Illek, M. Marounek, A. Nguyen Ngoc 2009 ,Feeding ruminally protected methionine to pre- and postpartum dairy cows: effect on milk performance, milk composition and blood parameters Institute of Animal Science, Praha-Uhřiněves, Czech Republic

Bauman, D.E., Griinari, J.M., 2001Regulation and nutritional manipulation of milk fat: low-fat milk syndrome,Livestock Production Science 70 15–29 (areview)

Dschaak, Christopher M., "Production Performance and Profles of Milk Faty Acids of Lactating Dairy Cows Fed Whole Safower Seed Containing High Fat and Low Fiber" (2009). All Graduate Theses and Dissertations. Paper 293

Garg, M.R., Sherasia, P.L. and Bhanderi, B.M., 2012. Effect of supplementing bypass fat with and without rumen protected choline chloride on milk yield and serum lipid profile in Jaffarabadi buffaloes. BUFFALO BULLEITN IBIC, KASETSART UNIVERSITY, PO BOX 1084 BANGKOK 10903, THAILAND, 31(2), p.91.

Gowda,N.K.S., A. Manegar1, A. Raghavendra, S. Verma, G. Maya,D.T. Pal, K.P. Suresh and K.T. Sampath, (2012)Effect of Protected Fat Supplementation to highyielding Dairy Cows in Field Condition , National Institute of Animal Nutrition and physiologybangalore-560 030, India (Received January 13,

Gulati, S.K., M.R. Garg and TW. Scott. 2005. Rumen protected protein and fat produced from oil seeds and meals by formaldehyde treatment; their role in ruminant production and product quality: A review. Aust. J. Exp. Agric. 45: 1189-1203.

Haryanto, B., 2014. Manipulating protein degradability in the rumen to support higher ruminant production. WARTAZOA. Indonesian Bulletin of Animal and Veterinary Sciences, 24(3).

Hassen A, Ebro A, Kurtu M and Treydte A C 2010: Livestock feed resources utilization and management as influenced by altitude in the Central Highlands of Ethiopia. Livestock Research for Rural Development. Volume 22, Article #229. Retrieved April 29, 2017, from Http://www2.luresext.edu/international/nutrconstraints.htm

Https://www.researchgate.net/publication/299854207Feeding_dairy_cattle_in_East_Africa_title?Enrichid=rgreq707b3adb51802455c74f285a2ba1ad5dxxx&enrichsource=y292zxjqywdlozi5otg1ndiwnztbuzozndgymtcwmdc5odq2ndnamtq2mdazmjgxmjm3mq%3D%3D&el=1_x&_esc=publicationcoverp

Hwang ,J. , Yun-Hee Chang1, J.H P ark, Soo Yeon Kim3, Haeyon Chung3, Eugene Shim4 and Hye Jin 2011 Dietary saturated and monounsaturated fats protect against acute acetaminophen hepatotoxicity by altering fatty acid composition of liver microsomal membrane in rats

Influxlipids,(2017)nderstanding-rumenprotected,http://www.influxlipids.com/ufat?Gclid=Cj0KEQjww7zhbrctopsj_c_wjzibeiqaj8il5omlj0w2zo22wydrpexv_qw_wbsewpt0eook9imfquaag Op8P8HAQ Accesed on April ,2017

Kalscheur, K.F. and Baldwin, V.I., BP & Kohn, RA, 2006. Milk production of dairy cows fed differing concentrations of rumen-degraded protein. J. Dairy Sci, 89, pp.249-259.

Muralidhar Karanam, «An improved protein extraction method for detecting ruminant material in feed using lateral flow device dipsticks», *BASE* [En ligne], Volume 15 (2011), numéro spécial 1, 25-29 URL : http://popups.ulg.ac.be/1780-4507/index.php?id=6830..

Khandaker, Z.H., Uddin, M.M., Sultana, M.N. and Peters, K.J., 2012. Effect of supplementation of mustard oil cake on intake, digestibility and microbial protein synthesis of cattle in a straw-based diet in Bangladesh. Tropical animal health and production, 44(4), pp.791-800.

Kirovski, D., Blond, B., Katić, M., Marković, R. And Šefer, D., 2015. Milk yield and composition, body condition, rumen characteristics, and blood metabolites of dairy cows fed diet supplemented with palm oil. Chemical and Biological Technologies in Agriculture, 2(1), p.6.

Lee I. Chiba (2014) Dairy Cattle Nutrition and Feeding .B. Fresh cows need special nutrition and feeding facilities to maximize their milking. Animal Nutrition Handbook. Section 15: ttp://www.ag.auburn.edu/~chibale/an15dairycattlefeeding.pdf

Leiva,* R. F. Cooke, A. P. Brandão, R. Marques,† and J. L. M. Vasconcelos.,2015. Effects of rumen-protected choline supplementation on metabolic and performance responses of transition dairy cows1 Department of Animal Production, São Paulo State University, Botucatu 18168-000, Brazil; and †Eastern Oregon Agricultural Research Center, Oregon State University, Burns 97720

Lock, A.L., Preseault, C.L., Rico, J.E., deland, K.E. and Allen, M.S., 2013. Feeding a C16: 0-enriched fat supplement increased the yield of milk fat and improved conversion of feed to milk. Journal of dairy science, 96(10), pp.6650-6659.

Lukuyu, B.A., Gachuiri, C.K., Lukuyu, M.N., Lusweti, C. And Mwendia, S., 2012. Feeding dairy cattle in East Africa.

Lusweti and Mwendia ,2012 Feeding dairy cattle in East Africa technical editors: Ben lukuyu and charles Gachuiri ompiled bycha rles Gachuiri, margaret lukuyu,

Mahima, Kumar V, Tomar SK, Roy D, Kumar M ,2015 , Effect of varying levels of formaldehyde treatment of mustard oil cake on rume fermentation, digestibility in wheat straw based total mixed diets in vitro Veterinary World 8(4); 551-555.

Martínez AL, Pérez M, Pérez LM, Carrión D, Garzón AI, Gómez G. Effect of dietary fat on the productive results of dairy ruminants. Rev Colomb Cienc Pecu 2013; 26:69-78.

Maurice L. Eastridge ,2014 Feeding Fat, in Moderation, to Dairy Cows Department of Animal Sciences .The Ohio State University

Mesfin, D., S. Bediye, A. Kehaliw, G. Kitaw and K. Nesha,2009. On-farm evaluation of lactating crossbred (Bos taurus x Bos indicus) dairy cows fed a basal diet of urea treated teff (Eragrostis tef) straw supplemented with escape protein source during the dry season in crop-livestock production system of north Shoa, Ethiopia. Livestock Research for Rural Development. 21 (5).

Muhammad Sarwar, A. S.-u.-N. 2003. Effect of Feeding Saturated Fat on Milk Production and Composition in Crossbred Dairy Cows. Department of Animal Nutrition, University of Agriculture, Faisalabad, Pakistan

Muller, L.2003, Fat supplementation with pasture-based systems. Penn state university (lmuller@psu.edu
Naik, P.K. 2013. Bypass fat in dairy ration-A review. Animal Nutrition and Feed Technology,13: 147-163.

Patton RS, Sorenson CE, Hippen AR .2004. Effects of dietary glucogenic precursors and fat on feed intake and carbohydrate status of transition dairy cows. J Dairy Sci 87:2122–2129

Pavkovych,S. Stakh V, Barna Kruzhel .2015 PROTECTED LIPIDS AND FATTY ACIDS IN CATTLEFEED RATIONS, Lviv National Agrarian University, Ukraine

Perfield, J. W., A. L. Lock, A. M. Pfeiffer, and D. E. Bauman. "Effects of amide-protected and lipid-encapsulated conjugated linoleic acid (CLA) supplements on milk fat synthesis." Journal of dairy science 87, no. 9 (2004): 3010-3016.

Pipat Lounglawan*, W.s , 2006 . The effect of ruminal bypass fat on milk yields and milk composition of lactating dairy cow

Rabiee, A.R., Breinhild, K., Scott, W., Golder, H.M., Block, E. And Lean, I.J., 2012. Effect of fat additions to diets of dairy cattle on milk production and components: A meta-analysis and meta-regression. Journal of dairy science, 95(6), pp.3225-3247.

Reynal, S.M. and GA Broderick. 2005. Effect of dietary level of rumen-degraded protein on production and nitrogen metabolism in lactating dairy cows. J. Dairy Sci. 88: 4045-4064.. Anim. Sci. 2003. Vol 16, No. 2 : 204-210) page 208

Shelke, S.K. and Thakur, S.S., 2011. Effect on the Quality of Milk and Milk Products in Murrah Buffaloes (Bubalus bubalis) Fed Rumen Protected Fat and Protein. International Journal of Dairy Science, 6(2), pp.124-133

Solomon , 2011. Current status of dairy cow feeding in the Ethiopian Central Highlands and some recommendations for promising technologies, ILRI internationallivestock Research Institute .

Strusińska, D. Minakowski, B. Pysera, J. Kaliniewicz   2006   Effects of fat-protein supplementation of diets for cowsin early lactation on milk yield and composition Department of Animal Nutrition and Feed Management, University of Warmia and Mazuria,Olsztyn, Poland

Taylor VJ, Beever DE & Wathes DC 2003 . Physiological adaptations to milk production that affect fertility in high yielding dairy cows. British Society of Animal Science Occasional Publication, vol 29, pp. 37–71. Nottingham, UK: Nottingham University

Tekeba E, Wurzinger M and Zollitsch W., 2014. Nutritional Limitations and Dairy Genotypes Interactions in Ethiopia.
AIJCSR, BOKU-University of Natural Resources and Life Sciences Vienna, Austria. 1(3): 125-137

Walli, T. K., and S. K. Sirohi 2004 ."Evaluation of heat treated (roasted) soybean on lactating cross bred cows." Project Report of the Collaborative Project between National Dairy Research. Research Institute, Karnal and American Soybean Association. New Delhi

Walli, T.K., 2005. Bypass protein technology and the impact of feeding bypass protein to dairy animals in tropics: A review. Indian J. Anim. Sci., 75: 135-142.

Weiss, W.P. and Pinos-Rodríguez, J.M., 2009. Production responses of dairy cows when fed supplemental fat in low-and high-forage diets. Journal of Dairy Science, 92(12), pp.6144 6155.

Weiner A,Ilona P, Agata G ,Krzysztof K,2015,Occurrence of animal-originconstituents in feeds ,Department of Hygiene of Animal Feedingstuffs, National Veterinary Research Institute, 24-100 Pulawy, Poland aweiner@piwet.pulawy.pl Received: September 1, 2014 Accepted: February 27, 2015

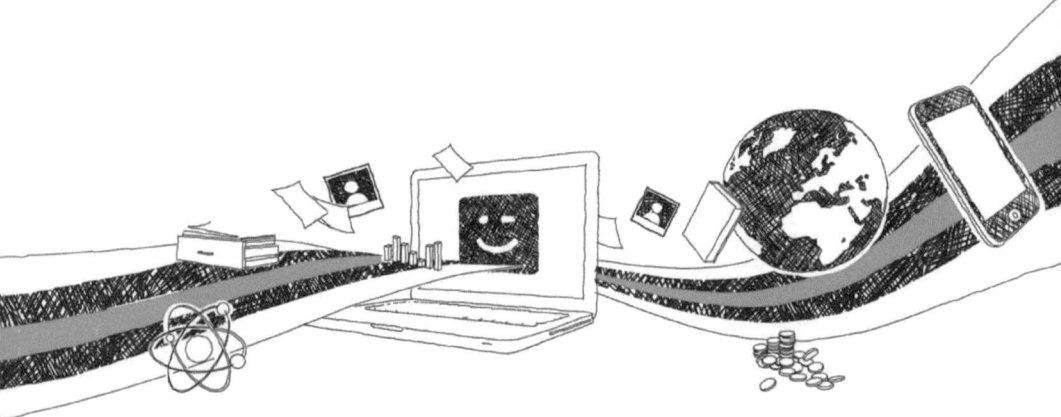
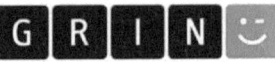